Table of Contents

There are many types of heart disease, and each one has its own symptoms and treatment. For some, lifestyle changes and medicine can make a huge difference in improving your health. For others, you may need surgery to make your ticker work well again.

Find out about some of the common types of heart disease and how to prevent them as well as how they're treated.

BREAKFAST

1. Oat Avocado-Berry Bars

Prep Time: 35 Minutes

Cook Time: 50 Minutes

Servings: 15

Ingredients

- Crust / Topping Ingredients
- Cooking spray
- 1 3/4 cups low-fat, low sugar granola
- 1 1/2 cups whole-wheat flour
- 2 tablespoon firmly packed brown sugar
- 1 teaspoon ground cinnamon
- 1/4 teaspoon salt
- 1/2 cup fat-free sour cream
- 2 tablespoon canola oil

Filling:

- 1/2 cup pitted, coarsely chopped dates

- 1/2 cup avocado
- 1 cup frozen, unsweetened blueberries
- 1 tablespoon grated orange zest
- 1 teaspoon cornstarch

Instructions

1. Preheat the oven to 350°F. Lightly spray a 13 x 9 x 2-inch baking pan with cooking spray.
2. Put the granola in a food processor. Pulse three times to break apart the large pieces (it should look like rolled oats). Transfer the granola to a large bowl. Stir in the flour, brown sugar, cinnamon, and salt until combined. Add the sour cream and oil.
3. Using a pastry blender or large fork, blend the mixture until it resembles pea-size crumbs.
4. Set aside one-half of the granola mixture. Press the other half into the baking pan to form a crust.
5. Bake the crust for 20 minutes, or until slightly browned. Transfer to a cooling rack. Let cool to room temperature.
6. Meanwhile, in a food processor, process the dates until smooth. Add the avocado, processing until

smooth. Add the blueberries, orange zest, and cornstarch, processing until smooth.

7. Spoon the filling onto the cooled crust. Use a spatula to spread it. Sprinkle the reserved granola mixture over the filling. Bake for 15 minutes, or until the topping is slightly browned and the filling is set.

8. Transfer the baking pan to a cooling rack. Let cool. Cut into 15 bars.

Prep Time: 15 Minutes

Cook Time: 35 Minutes

Servings: 4

Ingredients

- Cooking spray
- 4 6-inch corn tortillas
- 1 tablespoon canola oil

OR

- 1 tablespoon corn oil
- 1 medium red bell pepper (finely diced)

OR

- 1 medium green bell pepper (finely diced)
- 1/2 cup diced red onion
- 1 medium tomato (diced)
- 2 ounces fat-free cream cheese (cut into pieces)
- 2 large eggs
- 2 large egg whites

- 1 medium avocado (halved, pitted, mashed with a fork)
- 1/4 cup chopped, fresh cilantro (optional)
- 2 teaspoons chopped pickled jalapeños (drained)

Instructions

1. Preheat the oven to 400°F. Line a baking sheet with aluminum foil. Lightly spray the foil with cooking spray.
2. Arrange the tortillas in a single layer on the baking sheet. Lightly spray the tortillas with cooking spray. Bake for 6 to 7 minutes on each side, or until golden brown.
3. In a medium nonstick saucepan, heat the oil over medium-high heat, swirling to coat the bottom. Cook the bell pepper and onion for 5 to 7 minutes, or until the bell pepper is tender and the onion is soft, stirring occasionally. Cook the tomato for 2 to 3 minutes, or until it releases its liquid. Stir in the cream cheese. Cook the vegetable mixture for 2 to 3 minutes, or until the cream cheese has melted. Remove from the heat. Transfer the bell pepper mixture to a small bowl.

4. In a separate small bowl, whisk together the eggs and egg whites with a fork.

5. Wipe the pan with paper towels. Lightly spray the pan with cooking spray. Cook the egg mixture over medium-high heat, or until the eggs are scrambled, stirring constantly. Remove from the heat.

6. Spread the avocado over each tortilla. Top with the vegetable mixture and scrambled eggs. Garnish with the cilantro and jalapeños.

Prep Time: 45 Minutes

Cook Time: 50 Minutes

Servings: 5

Ingredients

Salsa:

- 2 cups chopped tomatoes (about 2 medium tomatoes)
- 1 medium avocado, halved, pitted, and diced (optional)
- 1 large ear of corn, husks and silk discarded, and kernels removed from the cob

OR

- 1 cup frozen whole-kernel corn, thawed and drained (optional)
- 1 to 2 medium fresh jalapeños, seeds and ribs discarded, finely chopped
- 2 tablespoons finely chopped red onion
- 2 tablespoons fresh lime juice
- Tostada Ingredients
- Cooking spray

- 5 6-inch corn tortillas
- 8 ounces ground skinless turkey breast
- 2 teaspoons chili powder
- 1 teaspoon ground cumin
- 1 teaspoon ground coriander
- 1 15.5-ounce can no-salt-added black beans, rinsed and drained
- 2 tablespoons water

Instructions

1. In a small bowl, stir together all the salsa ingredients. Set aside.
2. Preheat the oven to 400°F. Line a baking sheet with aluminum foil. Lightly spray the foil with cooking spray.
3. Place the tortillas on the baking sheet. Lightly spray the tortillas with cooking spray. Using a fork, pierce the tortillas a few times to prevent them from filling with air. Bake for 5 to 6 minutes on each side, or until golden brown.
4. Meanwhile, in a medium nonstick saucepan, cook the turkey, chili powder, cumin, and coriander over medium-high heat for 5 to 6 minutes, or until the

turkey is no longer pink, stirring occasionally to turn and break up the turkey.

5. Add the beans and water. Cook for 5 minutes, or until the beans are heated through. Using a potato masher. coarsely mash the beans. Remove from the heat.

6. To assemble the tostadas, spread the turkey mixture over each tortilla. Spoon the salsa over all.

Prep Time: 15 Minutes

Cook Time: 25 Minutes

Servings: 12

Ingredients

- Cooking spray (optional)
- 1 medium ripe avocado, halved, pitted, and mashed with a fork
- 1/2 cup sugar
- 1/2 cup fat-free milk
- 2 large eggs
- 1 teaspoon vanilla extract
- 2 cups all-purpose flour
- 2 teaspoons baking powder
- 1 teaspoon ground ginger
- 1/16 teaspoon salt
- 2 cups blueberries

Instructions

1. Preheat the oven to 375°F. Lightly spray a standard 12-cup muffin pan with cooking spray or line it with paper baking cups.
2. In a large bowl, stir together the avocado, sugar, milk, eggs, and vanilla.
3. In a medium bowl, stir together the flour, baking powder, ginger, and salt.
4. In two or three batches, stir the flour mixture into the avocado mixture until just moistened but no flour is visible. Don't overmix. Gently fold in the blueberries. Spoon the batter into the muffin cups.
5. Bake for 25 to 30 minutes, or until a wooden toothpick inserted in the center comes out clean and the muffins are golden brown, turning the pan once after 15 minutes of baking time.
6. Transfer the pan to a cooling rack. Let stand for 5 minutes.

Prep Time: 25 Minutes

Cook Time: 45 Minutes

Servings: 10

Ingredients

- 3 large ears of corn, husks and silk discarded, kernels cut off the cobs
- 2 large eggs
- 1 medium avocado, halved, pitted and coarsely mashed with a fork
- 3/4 cup all-purpose flour
- 1/4 cup fat-free milk
- 2 tablespoons chopped fresh chives
- 1 teaspoon baking powder
- 1/4 teaspoon salt
- 1/8 teaspoon pepper (freshly ground preferred)
- 1 1/2 teaspoons canola or corn oil and 1 1/2 teaspoons canola or corn oil, divided use
- Cooking spray

Instructions

1. In a medium bowl, stir together the corn, eggs, avocado, flour, milk, chives, baking powder, salt, and pepper.

2. In a large nonstick skillet, heat 1 1/2 teaspoons oil over medium-high heat, swirling to coat the bottom. Lightly spray a 1/4-cup measuring cup with cooking spray. Using the measuring cup, scoop up the avocado mixture and mound it in the skillet. Fit as many fritters as you can without overcrowding the skillet (about 5). Using a spatula that has been lightly sprayed with cooking spray, gently press down on the fritters.

3. Cook the fritters for 2 to 3 minutes, or until golden brown. Turn over. Using the spatula, gently press down on the fritters. Cook for 2 to 3 minutes, or until golden brown. Transfer to a large plate or platter lined with paper towels.

4. In the same skillet, still over medium-high heat, heat the remaining 1 1/2 teaspoons oil, swirling to coat the bottom. Repeat the cooking process with the remaining batter. Reduce the heat if the fritters are cooking too fast and starting to burn. Serve warm.

Prep Time: 15 Minutes

Cook Time: 25 Minutes

Servings: 4

Ingredients

- 3 ounces chicken, 3/4 cup vegetables, and 1 1/2 teaspoons feta
- 2 teaspoons olive oil
- 1 small onion, chopped
- 1 pound boneless, skinless chicken breasts, all visible fat discarded, cut into 1/2 x 2-inch strips
- 1/2 cup fat-free, low-sodium chicken broth
- 4 medium garlic cloves, minced
- 1 teaspoon ground cumin
- 1 teaspoon paprika
- 1/2 teaspoon ground turmeric
- 1/2 teaspoon pepper (coarsely ground preferred)
- 1/4 teaspoon salt
- 2 cups torn romaine lettuce
- 1 medium tomato, sliced, and 1 medium tomato, chopped, divided use

- 1/2 medium unpeeled cucumber, sliced, and 1/2 medium unpeeled cucumber, chopped, divided use
- 2 tablespoons crumbled low-fat feta cheese
- 2 tablespoons minced fresh Italian (flat-leaf) parsley

Instructions

1. Heat the oil in the pressure cooker on sauté. Cook the onion for 3 minutes, or until soft, stirring frequently. Add the chicken. Cook the chicken for 4 to 6 minutes, or until lightly browned, stirring frequently. Turn off the pressure cooker.

2. Stir in the broth, garlic, cumin, paprika, turmeric, pepper, and salt. Secure the lid. Cook on high pressure for 4 minutes. Quickly release the pressure.

3. Arrange as follows on a platter: the romaine, sliced tomato, and sliced cucumber. Using a slotted spoon, place the chicken on the cucumbers. Top with the remaining chopped cucumber and chopped tomato. Sprinkle with the feta and parsley.

Prep Time: 15 Minutes

Cook Time: 25 Minutes

Servings: 4

Ingredients

- 1/4 cup uncooked quinoa, rinsed and drained
- 2 medium tomatoes, chopped (about 2 cups)
- 1 cup no-salt-added frozen corn, thawed
- 1/2 medium avocado, pitted and diced
- 1/4 cup chopped green onions
- 1/2 cup chopped fresh cilantro (optional)
- Cooking spray
- 4 large eggs
- 1/8 teaspoon salt
- 1/4 teaspoon pepper
- Red hot-pepper sauce to taste (optional)

Instructions

1. Cook the quinoa according to the package directions. Remove from the heat.

2. Spoon the quinoa into four bowls. Top each with tomatoes, corn, avocado, green onions and cilantro.

3. Lightly spray a large skillet with cooking spray. Crack the eggs into the skillet. Sprinkle the salt and pepper over the eggs. Cook, uncovered, over medium-high heat for 3 to 4 minutes, or until the egg whites are set but the yolks are still runny. Using a spatula, carefully transfer one egg sunny side up into each of the bowls. Sprinkle with the hot sauce.

Prep Time: 35 Minutes

Cook Time: 50 Minutes

Servings: 6

Ingredients

For the Cheese and Vegetable Frittata:

- 6 large eggs
- 2 tablespoon whole-wheat flour
- 1 teaspoon baking powder
- 1/4 teaspoon black pepper
- 1 medium onion (about 1 cup), cut into 1/2 inch pieces
- 1 cup fresh or frozen spinach, cut into 1/2-inch pieces
- 1 cup red and/or green bell pepper, cut into 1/2-inch pieces
- 1 cup fresh mushrooms

OR

- 1 cup canned mushrooms
- 1 clove garlic (finely chopped)
- 2 tablespoon fresh basil leaves (finely chopped)
- 1/3 cup part-skim mozzarella cheese (shredded)

- Cooking spray

For the Fruit Salad:

- 2 peeled oranges, cut in half, then into 6-8 pieces, depending on their size
- 1 cup fresh green, red or purple grapes (use varieties without seeds), left whole
- 1 cup fresh or frozen strawberries, if fresh remove green top, sliced in half or quarters depending on their size
- 1 cup fresh or frozen mixed berries (blueberries, blackberries and/or raspberries)
- 2 tsp balsamic or white wine vinegar OR fresh or bottled lime or lemon juice OR pineapple and/or orange juice
- 2 teaspoon olive oil
- 2 Tbsp mint or basil leaves, left whole, removed from stems

Instructions

For the Cheese and Vegetable Frittata:

1. Preheat oven (regular or toaster oven) to broil setting.

1. In a large bowl, whisk eggs together until foamy, stir in the whole wheat flour, black pepper, and baking powder.
2. Using a heavy skillet with an ovenproof handle, coat the skillet with cooking spray and heat on medium.
3. Add the onion and cook until it starts to get soft, then add the spinach, bell pepper and mushrooms and cook for 2-3 minutes more.
4. Add the garlic and basil and cook for 1 minute. Stir to avoid burning these.
5. Add the egg mixture into the pan and stir to mix the vegetables with the eggs.
6. Cook for 5-6 minutes or until the egg mixture has set on the bottom and begins to set on top.
7. Add the shredded cheese and using the back of the spoon, push lightly under the eggs, so it won't burn in the oven.
8. Place pan into the oven and broil for 3-4 minutes until golden and fluffy.
9. Remove from pan, cut into 6 servings and serve.

For the Fruit Salad:

1. In a large bowl combine all fruit salad ingredients.
2. In a small covered jar shake the vinegar or juice with the olive oil to mix.

3. Add dressing to the fruit and toss to coat. If using frozen fruit toss very gently to avoid breaking them up too much.

Garnish with the fresh herbs, if available.

1. Serve with the frittata.

Prep Time: 35 Minutes

Cook Time: 50 Minutes

Servings: 4

Ingredients

- Cooking spray
- 1 1/3 cups liquid egg whites
- 1 15.5-ounce can no-salt-added black beans, rinsed and drained
- 4 6-inch whole-wheat tortillas (lowest sodium available)
- 2 medium avocados, sliced
- 1/4 cup hot sauce or salsa (lowest sodium available) (optional)

Instructions

1. Lightly spray a large skillet with cooking spray. Heat over medium heat.
2. Pour the egg whites into the skillet, stirring constantly with a rubber spatula to scramble. Cook until the eggs

are almost set. Add the beans, stirring until combined and heated through.

3. Microwave the tortillas on 100% power (high) for 45 seconds. (This makes them pliable and easier to roll.) Transfer to a work surface.
4. Spread the egg mixture in the center of each tortilla.
5. Top with the avocado and hot sauce.
6. For each burrito, fold two sides of the tortilla toward the center. Starting from the unfolded side closest to you, roll the burrito toward the remaining unfolded side to enclose the filling. Transfer with the seam side down to plates.

Prep Time: 40 Minutes

Cook Time: 60 Minutes

Servings: 4

Ingredients

For the Avocado Cream:

- 1 small avocado, halved, pitted, and coarsely chopped
- 1/2 cup fat-free or low-fat sour cream
- 2 tablespoons cold water
- 1 tablespoon chopped fresh cilantro

OR

- 1 teaspoon dried cilantro
- 1/2 teaspoon honey
- For the Black Beans
- 1 15.5-ounce can no-salt-added black beans, rinsed and drained
- 1 tablespoon chopped fresh cilantro

OR

- 1 teaspoon dried cilantro

- 1/2 teaspoon fresh lime juice
- 1/2 teaspoon canola or corn oil

For the Chicken Tostadas

- 1/2 cup fresh or frozen corn

OR

- 1/2 cup no-salt-added canned corn, rinsed and drained
- 1 medium Roma tomato, diced
- 3 tablespoons diced red onion
- 1 small jalapeño, seeds and ribs discarded, diced
- 1 medium garlic clove, minced

OR

- 3/4 teaspoon minced jarred garlic
- Pepper to taste
- 4 6-inch corn tortillas
- 4 ounces shredded cooked skinless chicken breast, cooked without salt, all visible fat discarded
- Handful fresh cilantro leaves, coarsely chopped

Instructions

For the Avocado Cream:

1. In a small bowl, stir together the avocado, sour cream, water, cilantro, and honey. With the back of a spoon, mash the mixture until combined and creamy.
2. For the Black Beans
3. In a food processor or blender, process the beans, cilantro, lime juice, and oil until smooth.

For the Chicken Tostadas

1. Preheat the oven to 350°F.
2. In a small bowl, stir together the corn, tomato, onion, jalapeño, garlic, and pepper.
3. Place the tortillas directly on the oven rack. Bake for 8 to 10 minutes, or until crisp. Transfer to a work surface.
4. Spread the bean mixture on the tortillas. Add the chicken. Spoon the tomato-corn salsa over the chicken. Top with a dollop of the avocado cream. Sprinkle with the cilantro leaves.

Prep Time: 30 Minutes

Cook Time: 1hrs 10 Minutes

Servings: 6

Ingredients

Baked Mozzarella Cheese Bites:

- Cooking spray
- 2 1/2 tablespoons cornstarch
- 1 1/2 cups whole-wheat or plain panko
- 2 large egg whites
- 2 tablespoons water
- 1/4 teaspoon pepper
- 6 low-fat mozzarella string cheese sticks (about 1 ounce each), each cut into 4 pieces

Easy Marinara Sauce:

- 1 1/2 cups no-salt-added crushed tomatoes
- 2 1/2 teaspoons dried Italian seasoning, crumbled
- 1/4 teaspoon pepper

Instructions

Baked Mozzarella Cheese Bites

1. Preheat the oven to 425°F. Line a large baking sheet with aluminum foil. Lightly spray the foil with cooking spray.
2. Put the cornstarch in a gallon-size resealable plastic bag. Put the panko in a second gallon-size resealable plastic bag. In a shallow dish, whisk together the egg whites, water, and pepper.
3. Add eight cheese pieces to the bag with the cornstarch, shaking to coat well. Dip the cheese pieces in the egg mixture, coating well. Transfer the cheese to the bag with the panko, shaking the bag until each cheese piece is well coated. Transfer to the baking sheet. Working in two batches, repeat with the remaining cheese.
4. Bake for 5 minutes, or until the cheese is melted.
5. Serve with the marinara sauce for dipping.

Easy Marinara Sauce

1. In a medium saucepan, over medium-high heat, cook the tomatoes, Italian seasoning, and pepper for 5 minutes, or until heated through, stirring frequently.

2. Simmer, covered, until ready to serve with the cheese
    bites.

Prep Time: 20 Minutes

Cook Time: 50 Minutes

Servings: 8

Ingredients

- 1 teaspoon canola oil

OR

- 1 teaspoon corn oil
- 1 medium onion (yellow preferred), diced
- 2 medium garlic cloves or 1 teaspoon jarred minced garlic (optional)
- 1 1/2 teaspoons ground cumin
- 1 1/2 teaspoons ground coriander
- 1 teaspoon ground cinnamon
- 1/2 teaspoon salt
- 1/4 teaspoon pepper
- 1 2-pound butternut squash, peeled, seeds and strings discarded, and chopped into 1-inch cubes (about 4 cups)

OR

- 20 ounces frozen butternut squash cubes

- 5 cups low-sodium vegetable broth

- 1 28-ounce can no-salt-added diced tomatoes

- 1 15-ounce can no-salt-added lentils

OR

- 3/4 cup dried lentils, sorted for stones and shriveled lentils, rinsed, and drained

- 3/4 cup chopped fresh cilantro

- 1 teaspoon grated lemon zest

Instructions

1. In a large pot or Dutch oven, heat the oil over medium-high heat, swirling to coat the bottom. Cook the onion for 3 minutes, or until soft, stirring frequently.

2. Stir in the garlic, cumin, coriander, cinnamon, salt, and pepper. Cook for 1 minute, or until the garlic and spices are fragrant. Stir in the butternut squash, broth, tomatoes, and lentils.

3. Bring to a boil. Reduce the heat to low. Simmer, covered, for 40 minutes, or until the lentils are tender. Sprinkle with the cilantro and lemon zest.

Prep Time: 34 Minutes

Cook Time: 45 Minutes

Servings: 4

Ingredients

- 1 teaspoon canola or corn oil
- 2 peeled apples, such as Fuji or Gala, chopped into 1-inch pieces
- 1 medium onion, chopped into 1-inch pieces
- 1/4 cup water, up to 1/4 cup water and 1/2 cup water, divided use
- 2 cups canned solid-pack pumpkin (not pie filling)
- 1 1/2 cups fat-free, low-sodium vegetable broth
- 1 tablespoon garam masala
- 1/4 teaspoon cinnamon

OR

- 1/4 teaspoon curry powder
- 1/2 cup fat-free milk
- 1/4 cup fat-free sour cream (optional)

- 1 tablespoon plus 1 teaspoon unsalted shelled pumpkin seeds, dry-roasted

Instructions

1. In a medium saucepan, heat the oil over medium-high heat, swirling to coat the bottom. Cook the apples and onion for 5 minutes, or until soft, stirring frequently.
2. Pour in 1/4 cup water. Cook, covered, for 7 minutes, or until the apples and onion are very soft, uncovering only once or twice to add 2 tablespoons of water as needed to prevent sticking (adding no more than 1/4 cup water total).
3. Gently stir in the pumpkin, broth, garam masala, cinnamon and remaining 1/2 cup water. Increase the heat to high and bring to a boil. Reduce the heat and simmer, covered, for 10 minutes.
4. In a food processor or blender (vent the blender lid), process the soup in batches for 10 to 15 seconds, or until slightly chunky. Carefully return to the pan.
5. Slowly pour in the milk, stirring until blended. Cook over medium heat for 30 seconds, or until heated through.

6. Garnish each serving with the sour cream and
   pumpkin seeds.

Prep Time: 34 Minutes

Cook Time: 45 Minutes

Servings: 4

Ingredients

- 1 cup soup and 1/2 cup salsa

Salsa:

- 1 medium peeled cucumber, finely diced (about 2 cups diced tomato)
- 2 medium tomatoes, seeded and diced (about 1 cup diced tomato)
- 1/2 cup chopped fresh cilantro
- 3 tablespoons fresh lime juice
- 2 tablespoons chopped red onion
- 1 to 2 tablespoons chopped fresh jalapeño, seeds and ribs discarded

Soup:

- Cooking spray
- 1 medium onion, chopped

- 3 medium zucchini, chopped (about 4 to 5 cups)
- 2 small garlic cloves garlic, crushed
- 1 1/2 cups fat-free, low-sodium vegetable broth
- 1 medium avocado, halved and pitted
- 1/2 cup low-fat buttermilk
- 2 tablespoons fresh lime juice
- 1/8 teaspoon salt
- 1/8 teaspoon pepper

Instructions

1. In a medium bowl, stir together all the salsa ingredients. Cover and refrigerate while making the soup.

2. Lightly spray a large skillet with cooking spray. Heat over medium-high heat. Cook the onion for 5 minutes, or until very soft. Stir in the zucchini and garlic. Cook for 5 minutes, or until the zucchini is tender, stirring constantly. Remove from the heat.

3. Transfer the zucchini mixture to a food processor or blender. Process for 30 seconds, or until mostly pureed. Add the remaining soup ingredients to the zucchini mixture. Process until smooth. Transfer the

soup to a container with a lid. Refrigerate until chilled or serve at room temperature.

4. At serving time, ladle the soup into bowls. Top each serving with the salsa.

5. To serve, ladle soup into 4 bowls. Top each bowl with the salsa, dividing it evenly.

Prep Time: 34 Minutes

Cook Time: 45 Minutes

Servings: 6

Ingredients

- 1/4 cup cider vinegar
- 3 tablespoons smooth low-sodium peanut butter
- 1 medium fresh jalapeño, seeds and ribs discarded, finely chopped
- 1 1/2 tablespoons hot water
- 2 teaspoons honey
- 1/4 teaspoon salt
- 1/8 teaspoon pepper, freshly ground preferred
- 1 14-ounce bag classic coleslaw mix
- 1 medium red or green bell pepper, thinly sliced
- 3 medium green onions, chopped (about ½ cup)
- 1/4 cup chopped unsalted peanuts

Instructions

1. In a large bowl, whisk together the vinegar, peanut butter, jalapeño, water, honey, and salt until combined.
2. Add the coleslaw mix, bell pepper, and green onions to the dressing.
3. Using tongs, toss the vegetables together with the dressing to coat.
4. Let stand for several minutes so the flavors blend. Sprinkle with the peanuts.

Prep Time: 15 Minutes

Cook Time: 60 Minutes

Servings: 4

Ingredients

- 2 tablespoons soy sauce
- 1 tablespoon water
- 1 tablespoon dry sherry

OR

- 1 tablespoon balsamic vinegar
- 1 tablespoon toasted sesame oil
- 1 large garlic clove, minced

OR

- 1 teaspoon bottled minced garlic
- 1 teaspoon minced peeled gingerroot (1 2-inch piece)
- 1 teaspoon white vinegar
- 1/2 teaspoon sugar substitute
- 4 6-ounce wild salmon fillets, skin removed
- 1 2-pound head cauliflower, coarsely chopped

- 1/2 medium onion, peeled and coarsely chopped
- 1 teaspoon canola or corn oil
- 1/8 teaspoon salt
- 1 cup chopped fresh cilantro
- 1 teaspoon sesame seeds
- 2 medium green onions, finely chopped

Instructions

1. In an ovenproof 8-inch square pan, whisk together the soy sauce, water, sherry, sesame oil, garlic, gingerroot, vinegar, and sugar substitute. Add the fish, turning to coat. Cover and refrigerate for at least 1 hour or up to 24 hours, turning occasionally. (Turn just once if you're refrigerating for only 1 hour.)

2. Put the cauliflower and onion in a large bowl. Stir to combine.

3. Transfer a small amount of the cauliflower mixture to a food processor or blender. Pulse until the mixture resembles couscous. (The key to achieving the right consistency is not overloading the food processor.) Transfer each batch of the processed mixture to a medium bowl until the rice is made. Cover and refrigerate until the fish is ready to bake.

4. When the fish has marinated, remove the pan from the refrigerator. Preheat the oven to 450°F.

5. Bake the fish and marinade for 10 to 12 minutes (depending on the thickness), or until the desired doneness, turning once halfway through. Remove from the oven. Transfer the fish to a baking sheet. Increase the heat to broil or turn on the broiler. Broil the fish for 2 to 4 minutes until browned on the outside, turning halfway through.

6. Meanwhile, in a large nonstick saucepan, heat the oil over medium-high heat, swirling to coat the bottom. Add the cauliflower mixture. Stir in the salt. Cook for 5 to 6 minutes, or until the cauliflower is tender, stirring frequently. Remove from the heat.

7. Stir in the cilantro. Transfer the cauliflower mixture to a platter.

8. Using a spatula, place the fish fillets on the cauliflower mixture.

9. Spoon the sauce from the baking pan over the fish. Sprinkle the sesame seeds and green onions over the sauce.

Prep Time: 34 Minutes

Cook Time: 55 Minutes

Servings: 6

Ingredients

- 1 1/2 cups pork and 3/4 cup brown rice
- 1 1/4 pound pork tenderloin (cut into 1/2-inch pieces)
- 1 tablespoon cornstarch
- 2 tablespoon white vinegar
- 1 tablespoon ketchup
- 2 teaspoons low-sodium soy sauce
- 2 teaspoons freshly grated gingerroot

OR

- 1/2 teaspoon ground ginger
- 3 cups peeled, thinly sliced carrots
- 2 cups snow peas (ends trimmed)
- 1/2 tablespoon canola oil
- 1/4 cup sliced scallions
- 1 20-ounce can pineapple chunks in own juice

- 3 1/2 cups cooked brown rice (from 1 cup uncooked brown rice), to serve

Instructions

1. Cut pork tenderloin into 1/2 inch pieces.
2. Add pork into a medium bowl or a large Ziploc bag along with cornstarch, vinegar, vinegar, ketchup, soy sauce, and ginger. Add all the pineapple juice from the can of pineapple chunks (about 1 cup) into the bowl/ Ziploc bag. (Reserve pineapple chunks for later use.) Mix together to combine and reserve until needed.
3. Thinly slice the carrots and trim the ends of the snow peas.
4. In a large skillet, warm oil over medium-high heat. Add carrots and stirring occasionally, cook about 5 minutes. Stir snow peas and pork into the mixture. Sauteeing and stirring constantly, cook until vegetables are soft and pork is fully-cooked, about 8 minutes.
5. Stir in reserved pineapple chunks and scallions. Cook 1 minute and remove from heat. Serve with brown rice.

Servings: 8

Ingredients

- 1 1/2 teaspoons canola or corn oil and 1 1/2 teaspoons canola or corn oil, divided use
- 2 pounds lean pork tenderloin, all visible fat discarded, cut into 1-inch pieces
- 4 medium ribs of celery, finely chopped
- 1 large onion, finely chopped
- 1 medium fresh jalapeño, seeds and ribs discarded, finely chopped (plus more for garnish, if desired)
- 2 tablespoons no-salt-added tomato paste
- 1 1/2 tablespoons chili powder
- 1 teaspoon ground cumin
- 1 teaspoon garlic powder
- 1/4 teaspoon ground pepper
- 3 cups water
- 1 14-5-ounce can no-salt-added diced tomatoes, drained
- 2 12-ounce packages frozen cooked winter squash puree, thawed

OR

- 2 15-ounce cans solid-pack pumpkin (not pie filling)
- 1 1 1/2-pound butternut squash, peeled, seeds removed, cut into 1-inch dice (about 2 cups)

OR

- 1 15-ounce cans solid-pack pumpkin (not pie filling)
- 2 14.5-ounce cans no-salt-added cannellini or white beans, rinsed and drained
- 1/2 cup chopped fresh cilantro (optional)
- 1/2 cup chopped green onions (optional)

Instructions

1. In a Dutch oven, heat 1 1/2 teaspoons oil over medium-high heat, swirling to coat the bottom. Cook the pork for 7 to 8 minutes, or until golden-brown, stirring occasionally. Transfer the pork to a small bowl.
2. Stir in the winter squash puree and pork. Increase the heat to high and bring the mixture to a boil. Reduce the heat and simmer, loosely covered, for 1 hour, or until the pork is tender.

3. Stir in the butternut squash and beans into the pork mixture. Increase the heat to high and bring to a boil. Reduce the heat and simmer, loosely covered, for 30 minutes, or until the butternut squash is tender.

4. Ladle the chili into bowls. Garnish with the cilantro, green onions, and jalapeño.

5. In the same pot, heat the remaining 1 1/2 teaspoons oil, swirling to coat the bottom. Cook the celery and onion for 5 minutes, or until slightly softened. Add the jalapeño, tomato paste, chili powder, cumin, garlic powder, and pepper. Cook for 1 minute, stirring constantly. Add the water and diced tomatoes, scraping the bottom of the pan to dislodge any browned bits.

Servings: 4

Ingredients

- 2 enchiladas
- 2 tablespoons canola or corn oil
- 1 tablespoon whole-wheat flour
- 1 cup fat-free, low-sodium chicken or vegetable broth
- 1 6-ounce can no-salt-added tomato paste
- 1 tablespoon chili powder
- 1 tablespoon brown sugar blend
- 1 teaspoon cumin
- 1/2 teaspoon onion powder
- 1/2 teaspoon garlic powder
- Cooking spray
- 4 medium zucchini
- 1/2 medium onion, diced
- 2 medium garlic cloves, minced
- 1/2 medium bell pepper (any color), diced
- 1/2 to 1 medium jalapeño, seeds and ribs discarded, diced (optional)

- 2 cooked boneless, skinless chicken breasts (about 4 ounces each), cooked without salt, all visible fat discarded, shredded
- 2 tablespoons chopped fresh cilantro
- 1/4 cup shredded low-fat cheddar cheese

Instructions

1. In a large skillet, heat the oil over medium heat, swirling to coat the bottom. Cook the flour, stirring constantly, until smooth.
2. Gradually stir in the broth, tomato paste, chili powder, brown sugar blend, cumin, onion powder, and garlic powder.
3. Bring to a boil over high heat, stirring occasionally. Reduce the heat and simmer for 5 to 10 minutes, or until thickened. Set aside.
4. Preheat the oven to 400°F. Lightly spray a 13 x 9 x 2-inch baking dish with cooking spray.
5. Halve the zucchini lengthwise. Scoop out the pulp, leaving a 1/4-inch border of the shell all the way around. Coarsely chop the pulp. Set aside.
6. Lightly spray a large skillet with cooking spray. Cook the onion, garlic, bell pepper, and jalapeño over

medium heat for 3 to 5 minutes, or until the onions are soft.

7. Stir in the chicken, cilantro, and reserved chopped zucchini. Cook for 3 minutes, or until the zucchini is tender.

8. Place the zucchini shells in the baking dish, cut side facing up. Using a pastry brush, lightly coat the inside of each zucchini shell with the enchilada sauce.

9. Spoon the chicken mixture into each zucchini shell. Spoon the remaining enchilada sauce over the chicken mixture. Sprinkle with the cheese.

10. Bake for 40 to 45 minutes, or until the cheese is melted and the zucchini shells are tender when pierced with a fork.

Servings: 6

Ingredients

- Cooking spray
- 4 medium zucchini, chopped (about 8 cups)
- 12 ounces whole-wheat spaghetti
- 2 cups tightly packed fresh basil, spinach, arugula, or mint
- 1 garlic clove, minced

OR

- 1 teaspoon jarred minced garlic
- 2 tablespoons unsalted walnuts or almonds
- 2 tablespoons fat-free, low-sodium chicken broth and 1 to 2 tablespoons fat-free, low-sodium chicken broth as needed
- 1 1/2 tablespoons extra-virgin olive oil or canola oil
- 1 1/2 tablespoons shredded or grated Parmesan cheese
- 1/4 teaspoon salt
- 1/8 teaspoon pepper

Instructions

1. Lightly spray a large skillet with cooking spray. Cook the zucchini over medium-high heat for 10 to 12 minutes, or until tender.

2. Meanwhile, prepare the pasta using the package directions, omitting the salt. Drain in a colander, reserving 1/4 cup pasta water.

3. In a food processor or blender, process the basil, garlic, walnuts, 2 tablespoons broth, oil, Parmesan, salt, pepper, and 2 cups zucchini for 1 minute, or until well blended. Add 1/2 tablespoon broth for a thinner consistency. Process for 30 seconds. Repeat until the desired consistency.

4. In a large bowl, stir together the pasta, pesto, and 1 tablespoon reserved pasta water. One tablespoon at a time, add the remaining pasta water until the desired consistency.

5. Top with the remaining zucchini.

21. Sautéed Zucchini, Tomato and Chickpea Ragout

Servings: 6

Ingredients

- 2 medium zucchini (chopped)
- 3 yellow squash (chopped)
- 28 oz. canned, no-salt-added, or, low-sodium tomatoes (crushed)
- 6 cups Chickpea Salad with Tomatoes and Cucumber
- 1 tsp. ground cumin
- 1/4 tsp. ground black pepper
- 3 cup whole-wheat couscous

Instructions

1. Spray a large sauté pan with cooking spray. Add chopped zucchini and cook over medium-high heat. Stirring occasionally with spatula, cook until zucchini are soft, about 5 minutes.

2. Add tomatoes, Chickpea Salad, cumin, and black pepper. Stir and bring to a boil. Once boiling, cover

with lid or foil. Reduce heat to low so mixture is simmering. Let ragout simmer 15 minutes.

3. Meanwhile, make couscous according to package directions (omitting the salt and fat).

4. Serve ragout over couscous.

Servings: 4

Ingredients

- Cooking spray
- 1 pound boneless, skinless chicken breasts, all visible fat discarded, cooked, cooled, and shredded
- 1 15.5-ounce can no-salt-added black beans, rinsed and drained
- 10 ounces frozen whole-kernel corn, thawed
- 1 15.25-ounce can no-salt-added corn, rinsed and drained
- 1 teaspoon chili powder and 2 teaspoons chili powder, divided use
- 12 6-inch whole-wheat or corn tortillas, warmed
- 1 14.5-ounce can no-salt-added tomato sauce
- 1/2 cup fat-free sour cream

Instructions

1. Preheat the oven to 400°F. Lightly spray a baking dish with cooking spray.

2. Put the chicken in a large bowl. Stir in the beans, corn, and 1 teaspoon chili powder.

3. Put six tortillas on a large cutting board or clean, flat surface. Spoon about 1 1/2 tablespoons of the chicken mixture down the center of the tortillas, stopping about 2 inches from the edges. Roll up and place with the seam side down in the baking dish, securing with a toothpick if desired.

4. In a small bowl, stir together the remaining 2 teaspoons chili powder, tomato sauce, and sour cream. Spoon over the tortillas.

5. Bake for 15 to 20 minutes, or until heated through.

Servings: 4

Ingredients

- 2 medium unpeeled zucchinis, grated with a box grater (about 3 cups)
- 1 small shallot, minced (about 1/4 cup)
- 2 large eggs, lightly beaten using a fork
- 1/2 cup all-purpose flour
- 1/4 cup shredded Parmesan cheese
- 1 1/2 teaspoons chopped, fresh thyme
- 1 teaspoon baking powder
- 1 teaspoon black pepper
- 1 teaspoon canola or corn oil and 1 teaspoon canola or corn oil, divided use
- 1/4 cup fat-free, plain Greek yogurt

Instructions

1. In a large bowl, stir together the zucchini, shallot, eggs, flour, Parmesan, thyme, baking powder, and pepper until well combined.

2. In a large nonstick skillet, heat 1 teaspoon oil over medium heat, swirling to coat the skillet. Place eight 1/8-cup mounds of the zucchini mixture in the skillet. Using the back of the measuring cup or a spoon, gently press down on the mounds, spreading them to make pancakes about 1/2-inch thick and 2 1/2 inches in diameter. Cook for 3 to 4 minutes on each side, or until golden brown all over. Transfer the pancakes to a plate. Cover to keep warm. Repeat with the remaining 1 teaspoon oil and zucchini mixture.

3. Let the pancakes cool for 5 minutes. Just before serving, top each pancake with a dollop of the yogurt.

Servings: 4

Ingredients

Catfish:

- Cooking spray
- 1 1/2 teaspoons paprika
- 1 teaspoon dried thyme, crumbled
- 1/2 teaspoon garlic powder
- 1/2 teaspoon onion powder
- 1/2 teaspoon cayenne
- 1/4 teaspoon pepper
- 4 catfish fillets (about 4 ounces each) or other mild white fish, such as tilapia or trout
- 1 tablespoon canola or corn oil

Collard Greens:

- 1 tablespoon canola or corn oil
- 1/2 small onion, thinly sliced
- 1 teaspoon bottled minced garlic
- 1 bunch collard greens, tough stems discarded, sliced into 1-inch pieces

- 1 slice uncured, nitrate-free Canadian bacon (lowest sodium available), cooked and diced
- 2 tablespoons water
- 1 tablespoon cider vinegar
- 1 teaspoon sugar
- 1/2 teaspoon crushed red pepper flakes

Instructions

Catfish:

1. Preheat the oven to 425°F. Lightly spray a 13 x 9 x 2-inch baking dish with cooking spray.
2. In a shallow bowl, whisk together the paprika, thyme, garlic powder, onion powder, cayenne, pepper and 1 tablespoon oil. Using your fingertips, gently press half of the mixture so it adheres to the fish. Turn over the fish. Repeat the process. Transfer the fish to the baking dish.
3. Bake for 15 minutes, or until the fish flakes easily when tested with a fork.
4. Serve the fish on the greens.

Collard Greens

1. In a large skillet, heat 1 tablespoon oil over medium heat, swirling to coat the bottom. Cook the onion for 3 minutes, or until soft, stirring occasionally. Add the garlic. Cook for 30 seconds, stirring constantly.
2. Stir in the greens, Canadian bacon, water, vinegar, sugar, and red pepper flakes.
3. Cook, covered, for 20 minutes, or until the greens are tender.

Servings: 4

Ingredients

- 3 ounces chicken, 2 tablespoons dipping sauce, and 1 zucchini

Chicken:

- 8 large green onions, coarsely chopped
- 2 medium fresh jalapeños, seeds and ribs discarded (optional)
- 4 medium garlic cloves
- 4 sprigs of fresh thyme
- 2 tablespoons honey
- 2 tablespoons fresh lime juice and 2 tablespoons fresh lime juice, divided use
- 1 tablespoon ground allspice
- 1 tablespoon cider vinegar
- 1 teaspoon ground cinnamon
- 1 teaspoon ground ginger
- 1 to 2 tablespoons water, as needed, and 1 to 2 tablespoons water, as needed, divided use

- 4 boneless, skinless chicken breasts (about 4 ounces each), all visible fat discarded
- Cooking spray
- 1/4 teaspoon black pepper
- 1/8 teaspoon salt
- 1 medium avocado, halved, pitted, and coarsely chopped
- 1/4 cup fat-free sour cream
- Zucchini Ingredients:
- 4 medium zucchini
- 1/2 cup plain or whole-wheat panko (Japanese-style bread crumbs)
- 1/4 cup shredded Parmesan cheese

OR

- 1/4 cup grated Parmesan cheese
- 1 tablespoon canola or corn oil
- 1/2 teaspoon dried Italian seasoning, crumbled
- 1/8 teaspoon salt

Instructions

1. In a food processor or blender, process the green onions, jalapeños, and garlic for 30 seconds, or until finely chopped. Add the thyme, honey, 2 tablespoons lime juice, the allspice, vinegar, cinnamon, and ginger. Process until smooth. Add 1 to 2 tablespoons of water if the marinade is too chunky and process until smooth.

2. Put the chicken in a large shallow dish. Add the marinade, turning to coat. Cover and refrigerate for 4 to 24 hours, turning occasionally.

3. When the chicken is ready, lightly spray the grill rack with cooking spray. Preheat on medium high.

4. Drain the chicken, discarding the marinade. Using paper towels, wipe most of it off the chicken. Sprinkle the pepper and salt over the chicken. Grill for 6 to 8 minutes on each side, or until it registers 165°F on an instant-read thermometer. Transfer the chicken to a plate. Cover with aluminum foil.

5. Cut each zucchini crosswise into 1/4-inch slices without cutting all the way through in a hasselback cut. (It's OK if you cut all the way through and break the zucchini. Just proceed as directed.) Gently fan the zucchini to open.

6. Place a double layer of aluminum foil on the grill. Make a large "boat" of foil to snugly hold the zucchini so they don't move around. Grill the zucchini without turning for 15 minutes, or until golden brown and almost tender.

7. In a small bowl, stir together the remaining zucchini ingredients. Sprinkle the panko mixture over the zucchini. Grill for 1 to 2 minutes. Remove from the grill.

8. Meanwhile, in a medium bowl, using an immersion, or handheld, blender, puree the avocado, sour cream, and the remaining 2 tablespoons lime juice until smooth. Add the remaining 1 to 2 tablespoons of water if the sauce is too thick. (You can also process the sauce in a food processor or blender until smooth.)

9. Serve the zucchini and sauce with the chicken.

Servings: 6

Ingredients

- 1 pound bottom round beef roast (cut into 1-inch cubes)
- 1 large russet potato, cut into 1/2-inch dice (about 2 cups)
- 1/4 cup all-purpose flour
- 1 medium sweet potato, cut into 1/2-inch dice (about 2 cups)
- 2 cups peeled, thinly sliced carrots
- 1 10-ounce package frozen pearl onions
- 1 14.5-ounce can no-salt-added diced tomatoes
- 1 14.5-ounce can fat-free, low-sodium beef broth
- 1 cup water
- 3/4 teaspoon dried thyme
- 1/2 teaspoon ground pepper
- 1 10-ounce package frozen peas
- 2 tablespoons dried parsley

Instructions

1. Add the beef, russet potato, and flour to a 4- to 6-quart slow cooker, stirring well to combine.

2. Add the sweet potato and carrots to the slow cooker. Top with the onions, tomatoes, broth, water, thyme, and pepper.

3. Cook, covered, for 10 to 12 hours on low heat or 5 to 6 hours on high heat. Just before serving, quickly stir in the peas and parsley. Re-cover. Cook for 5 to 10 minutes.

Servings: 4

Ingredients

- 1/2 cup tightly packed fresh cilantro
- 1/2 cup 100% orange juice (juice from 1 medium orange)
- 2 medium green onions, coarsely chopped
- 1/4 cup fresh lemon juice (from 1 to 2 medium lemons)
- 1/4 cup fresh lime juice (from 2 to 3 medium limes)
- 8 medium garlic cloves
- 1 teaspoon ground cumin
- 1 teaspoon dried oregano, crumbled
- 1 1/4 pounds pork tenderloin, all visible fat discarded
- 1 1/2 tablespoons canola or corn oil and 1 1/2 teaspoons canola or corn oil, divided use
- 1/8 teaspoon pepper and 1/8 teaspoon pepper (freshly ground preferred), divided use
- 1/8 teaspoon salt

- 2 ripe plantains, peeled and cut diagonally into slices about 1/2-inch thick
- Cooking spray

Instructions

1. In a food processor or blender, process the cilantro, orange juice, green onions, lemon juice, lime juice, garlic, cumin, and oregano. Process for about 1 minute, or until smooth. Transfer the marinade to a large shallow dish, reserving 1/4 cup. Add the pork, turning to coat. Cover and refrigerate for 2 to 24 hours, turning occasionally.
2. About 30 minutes before the pork is ready to grill, preheat the oven to 450°F and preheat the grill on medium high.
3. In a large bowl, whisk together 1 1/2 tablespoons oil, 1/8 teaspoon pepper, and the salt until combined. Add the plantain slices, turning to coat.
4. Cover a large baking sheet and two smaller ones with aluminum foil. Lightly spray all three sheets with cooking spray. Arrange the plantains in a single layer on the baking sheets. Bake for 15 minutes. Remove from the oven.

5. Turn over the plantains. Bake for 10 to 15 minutes, or until the plantains are crisp and caramelized on the outer edges. Watch carefully so they don't burn.

6. Meanwhile, drain the pork, gently wiping off most of the marinade. Discard the marinade.

7. Sprinkle the remaining 1/8 teaspoon pepper over the pork. Using a basting brush, brush the remaining 1 1/2 teaspoons oil over the pork. Transfer to the grill.

8. Grill the pork for 15 to 20 minutes, or until the thickest part of the pork reaches an internal temperature of 145°F, turning every few minutes.

9. Transfer the pork to a cutting board. Let stand for at least 5 minutes. Cut into slices. Transfer to a large platter. Spoon the reserved marinade over the pork. Serve with the plantains.

Servings: 4

Ingredients

- 4 medium sweet potatoes (thoroughly washed)
- 1 pound boneless, skinless chicken breasts
- 2 teaspoon extra virgin olive oil
- 1/2 teaspoon black pepper
- Cooking spray
- 1/2 medium white or yellow onion (diced)
- 3/4 cup frozen corn (thawed, drained)
- 15 ounces canned, low-sodium black beans
- juice of 1 lime
- 1 tsp no-calorie sweetener, granulated, 1 packet
- 1 teaspoon cumin
- 1 teaspoon chili powder
- 1/2 teaspoon garlic powder
- 1/2 teaspoon dried oregano
- 2 tablespoon water
- 2 tablespoon reduced-fat pepper jack cheese

Instructions

1. Preheat oven to 400.

2. Pierce each sweet potato all around with a fork. Place potatoes on a baking sheet and bake for 1 hour until potatoes pierce easily with a fork.

3. While potatoes are baking, rub chicken breasts with olive oil and place in a baking dish, sprinkle with pepper. Bake in the same oven as the potatoes in preheated oven for 20-25 minutes until chicken is cooked through. Remove chicken from the oven and let cool. Once cooled, shred chicken gently with a fork and set aside.

4. Spray a large skillet with cooking spray. Over medium heat, sauté onion 2-3 minutes until translucent. Stir in corn and beans stirring occasionally until heated through, approximately 3-5 minutes. Gently add chicken, lime juice, no-calorie sweetener, cumin, chili powder, garlic powder, oregano, and water. Stir until well blended and cook until mixture is warmed through.

5. Carefully remove potatoes from oven and slice open lengthwise (be careful of steam!). Add ¼ of bean and chicken mixture to each potato and top with cheese. Return to oven until cheese is melted.

29. Rosemary Balsamic Roasted Vegetables

Servings: 8

Ingredients

- Cooking spray
- 1/2 pound Brussels sprouts, brown ends trimmed off and cut in half
- 1/2 medium cauliflower (cut into florets)
- 4 medium carrots (sliced)
- 1/2 pound turnips (peeled, cut into 1/2-inch cubes)
- 1/2 pound beets (peeled, cut into 1/2-inch cubes)
- 1/3 pound sweet potatoes (peeled, cut into 3/4-inch cubes, optional)
- 3 tablespoons balsamic vinegar
- 3 teaspoons extra-virgin olive oil
- 2 teaspoons no-calorie sweetener (granulated)
- 2-3 tablespoons fresh, chopped rosemary

OR

- 2-3 teaspoons dried rosemary
- 2 medium garlic cloves, minced
- 1 teaspoon onion powder
- 1/2 teaspoon pepper

- 1/4 teaspoon salt

Instructions

1. Preheat the oven to 375°F.
2. Lightly spray 13 x 9 x 2-inch baking dish with cooking spray.
3. Place all the vegetables in a large bowl.
4. In a small bowl, whisk together the vinegar, oil, no-calorie sweetener, rosemary, garlic, onion powder, pepper and salt. Pour over the vegetable mixture, tossing to coat.
5. Pour the vegetable mixture into the baking dish. Bake for 30 to 35 minutes, stirring once, or until all the vegetables are tender when easily pierced with a fork.

Servings: 8

Ingredients

- 1 Tbsp. extra virgin olive oil
- 4 clove fresh, minced garlic

OR

- 4 tsp. jarred, minced garlic
- 1 small onion (chopped)
- 1 1/2 cups fresh, chopped kale (about 3 leaves), cut into bite-size pieces, stems discarded

OR

- 1 1/2 cups frozen spinach (thawed)
- 2 1/2 cups eggplant or summer squash, (about 1 small eggplant or 2 squash), cut into 1/2-inch cubes
- 1 1/2 cups tomatoes (diced)

OR

- 14.5 oz. canned, no-salt-added tomatoes (diced)
- 1 lb. extra-lean, ground beef or turkey, 95% lean or more

- 2 cups white mushrooms (sliced)
- 1 cup low-sodium, or, no-salt-added cannellini beans (drained, rinsed)
- 3/4 tsp. black pepper (divided use)
- 2 tsp. dried, salt-free herbs, Italian blend, divided use
- 1/2 cup low-moisture, part-skim mozzarella (shredded)
- 1/2 tsp. crushed red pepper
- 3 Tbsp. red wine vinegar
- 1/2 cup low-fat ricotta cheese
- 9 whole-grain sheets lasagna noodles
- 1 Tbsp. no-salt-added tomato paste
- 8 oz. canned, no salt added tomato sauce

Instructions

1. Preheat oven to 350° F.
2. Cook lasagna noodles according to package directions; omitting salt, butter and oil.
3. In a saucepan, heat oil. Add garlic and onion and cook over medium heat for about 4 minutes. Add kale (or spinach), tomatoes and eggplant (or squash) and pepper and cook 3 minutes. Turn up heat to medium-high, add ground beef or turkey and cook until meat

browns slightly and liquid is absorbed. Add mushrooms, beans, vinegar, tomato paste, and tomato sauce. Stir in red pepper flakes, 1 teaspoon dried herbs, ½ teaspoon of pepper. Simmer for 15 to 20 minutes, stirring occasionally.

4. Mix together mozzarella and 1 teaspoon dried herbs.

5. In a 9x13 ovenproof dish, place 3 lasagna sheets, one third of lasagna filling and half of ricotta in small clumps. Repeat placing the lasagna sheets, filling and ricotta step. Top with 3 more lasagna sheets, remaining filling and top with mozzarella mixture. Bake for 30 minutes.